Survive
CRNA School

A GUIDE TO SUCCESS AS A NURSE
ANESTHESIA STUDENT

Chris Mulder, CRNA, MSN

Contents

About the Author   5

PART 1: GET INTO CRNA SCHOOL   9

    INTRODUCTION   11

    STEP 1
    Get into nursing school   13

    STEP 2
    Work as a nurse in the ICU/ER   17

    STEP 3
    Get your CCRN   19

    STEP 4
    Take the GRE   21

    STEP 5
    Get Letters of Recommendation   23

    STEP 6
    Observe a CRNA   25

    STEP 7
    Apply to CRNA School   27

    STEP 8
    Nail the Interview   29

PART 2: SURVIVE CRNA SCHOOL   33

    INTRODUCTION   35

    CHAPTER ONE
    You're In! Now You Can Relax
    (Well, if You Have Some Xanax)   37

    CHAPTER TWO
    Getting Your Textbooks   43

CHAPTER THREE
Finding a Way to Pay for it 47

CHAPTER FOUR
Study Smarter, Not Harder 53

CHAPTER FIVE
The Classmate Advantage 61

CHAPTER SIX
Setting Up Before Cases 65

CHAPTER SEVEN
Big Pimpin' (Working With Preceptors) 73

CHAPTER EIGHT
Maintaining Confidence While Getting
the Most Out of Your Clinical Time 81

CHAPTER NINE
Coming to Terms With Your
New Hectic Schedule 87

CHAPTER TEN
Staying Off the Radar 93

CHAPTER ELEVEN
Preparing for the Unexpected 95

CHAPTER TWELVE
The Pre-op Interview and Post-op Report 99

CHAPTER THIRTEEN
Working With Others 103

CHAPTER FOURTEEN
Getting Certified and Finding a Job 107

CHAPTER FIFTEEN
Don't Stop Believing 113

About the Author

Growing up, I never knew I wanted to be a nurse anesthetist. Hell, I'd never even heard of it and probably couldn't pronounce it if I had. Just like most of my friends, I wanted to be a baseball player. Don't worry...of course I had a back-up career. I could always become an astronaut if things didn't work out as planned. After graduating high school, reality came crashing down all around me. I spent two years drifting through life at my local community college searching for my purpose in this world.

When I transferred to the nearest state university, I was forced to finally suck it up and make a decision. I've always liked to write, which is why I chose to obtain a degree in English. Unfortunately, someone forgot to tell me that I would eventually need to make a living. I'm sure there are some decent jobs an English graduate can get, but I couldn't find them. If you're not Stephen King or J.K. Rowling, it can be very difficult to make any real money in that field.

After spending a couple of years in a cubicle, selling things that people didn't want, I decided it was time to make a change. A friend suggested that I look into nurse anesthesia as a possible option, so I decided to check it out. This was the first I'd heard of it, and I thought she was pulling my leg. I spent several weeks researching the profession and the requirements to make it happen. Since my degree was in English, you can probably imagine the amount of pre-requisites I had to catch up on to get into nursing school.

I was fortunate enough to get into an accelerated BA/BS to BSN program on my first application. After nursing school, I started working as an RN in a Medical ICU. This experience only fortified my passion to become a CRNA. I loved titrating medications, making independent decisions, and helping patients and families get through difficult times. After 3 years, I finally managed to work my way into CRNA School. I had hoped to get accepted quicker, but I think I needed that time to be truly prepared for what I was about to get myself into.

CRNA School was the most difficult challenge I've ever had to endure. It tested me mentally and physically, and there were many times that I questioned whether I made the right decision. I'm glad I hung in there, because I really enjoy what I do now. I currently work at a level I trauma center taking care of all types of patients in almost all types of cases. On a few rare occasions, I get to take care of a healthy patient. But most of them are very sick with several comorbidities.

When I look back, it seems like just yesterday that I first stepped foot into the hospital as a nurse anesthesia student. At the same time, it seems like ages ago. I'm thankful for every difficult day I've gone through ever since deciding to become a CRNA. It has made me the person I am today, and I wouldn't change a thing. On second thought, I guess I could have done without a select few of those lectures!

PART 1

GET INTO CRNA SCHOOL

INTRODUCTION

If you've already been accepted into CRNA school, feel free to skip ahead to the next section. If you are considering the profession or are trying to get into a program, then this information is for you.

So you want to be a CRNA? It's a great profession and one in which you can make a very good living. However, the road that's required to get to that final destination is a long and grueling one. You will be tested every step of the way. But if you're willing to put in the time and effort, it can be extremely rewarding. Let's start from the beginning as though you had no medical background at all. After all, that's where I started from!

STEP 1
Get into nursing school

As I mentioned before, there is no easy step to becoming a CRNA, and this one is no exception. To get into either an RN or BSN program, a specific set of pre-requisite courses must first be completed. This may take you a year or longer depending on how determined you are. Here are some of the common pre-requisites:

- Anatomy and Physiology 1 (plus a lab course)
- Anatomy and Physiology 2 (plus a lab course)
- Algebra, Statistics (or some type of math course)
- Microbiology (plus a lab course)
- Sociology, Psychology (or similar)
- English

Of course, these may vary by program, but at least you have an idea of what's in front of you now. If you're serious about becoming a nurse, make sure you do well in these courses. You want to have a good GPA when it comes time to apply. Most schools have a minimum GPA required to get in (e.g. 2.8). But you will need much higher than the minimum to get into most places. These programs are extremely competitive, and they often have wait lists because of the high number of applicants. You probably want to shoot for a GPA of at least 3.5 or higher.

In addition to the pre-requisites, most schools will have you complete some kind of entrance exam, such as the TEAS. You will likely have to get a background check done, immunizations, a physical, drug screen, and CPR certification. If you decide to apply for admission directly into a BSN program, general studies courses will also be required, usually the equivalent of 2 years. You could always get your associate's degree to become an RN, and then continue into an RN to BSN program. Keep in mind that you will eventually need your BSN if you want to get into CRNA School.

Another option to getting your nursing degree is by attending a school that offers a Bachelor's to BSN program. In this case, you would have already received a bachelor's degree in another field. Since you have already competed most of the general studies requirements, these programs are usually accelerated, with most offering degree completion in 2 years or less.

Getting a bad grade in one class may ruin your chances of getting into many nursing schools. If this happens, most schools offer an option for "grade forgiveness." In this case, you would retake the class in an attempt for a better grade. If you do well, then the other grade drops off. For example, let's say you got a D in Biology. You retake the class, get an A, and the D gets forgiven. While the D will still show up on your transcript, it will not be calculated into your GPA.

Grade forgiveness is an option that is usually only available for classes in which you got a D or F. However, it is possible to do it if you got a C. Not every school will offer this, but it wouldn't hurt to check. You may have to petition the Dean or the President to make a C go away with a class retake. This is what I had to do when I got a C in Anatomy and Physiology 2. I thought the world was going to come to an end. But it didn't. I let the wave of depression pass over me before getting back to achieving my goal. I took the class again the next semester, and this time, I got an A!

If you get a poor grade or don't get in on your first try, don't spend time feeling sorry for yourself. Figure how to fix it to improve your chances of getting in next time. The important thing is to be tenacious and not give up.

STEP 2
Work as a nurse in the ICU/ER

The minimum requirement for admission into CRNA School is 1 year of experience in the ICU or ER. However, most programs require that you have at least 2 years of experience. Not all schools will accept ER experience either, so you might want to play it safe and get into the ICU as soon as possible.

Some people think that it is important to get many years of floor nursing under your belt before moving on to the ICU. However, I think a new graduate nurse can work in the ICU and hold their own just fine. This is how I did it, right after graduation. In a way, I think it is easier to start in the ICU before you get used to the world of floor nursing. They are extraordinarily different places to work in.

While in the ICU, don't be shy. Try to get as many experiences under your belt as possible. Offer to take care of the difficult patients with lots of drips and co-morbidities. Volunteer to start IVs for your co-workers and stay close to those who can teach you a thing or two.

Make the respiratory therapists your friends and have them show you how things work with the ventilator. Master ABGs and start to study up on your meds at a more molecular level. Start to think of your time in the ICU as on-the-job training for CRNA school. You will be happy you did when it comes time to interview and your first day in clinicals.

STEP 3
Get your CCRN

Although this isn't a requirement for most programs, it will look really good in a pool of hundreds of applicants. Spend at least a year before taking this exam, and study as much as you can beforehand. Not only will it help you get into CRNA School, but the information you'll learn will provide some value as an anesthesia provider.

Aside from gaining a great deal of knowledge, getting your CCRN will often get you a small pay raise in many places. Also, they will usually pay for your exam fee. Your fellow nurses will see that designation and see that you are someone who knows their stuff.

There are tons of places that offer preparation for the CCRN examination, such as CCRN Review Online or apps like CCRN Adult Exam Prep. You can also just do a search online and get tons of options

STEP 4
Take the GRE

This is a required test for most schools, though some will want the GMAT instead. Get a study guide and work through it before taking the exam. The minimum required score is usually around 300. This is a combined score derived from how well you did on the verbal section and the quantitative section.

Again, 300 is often just the minimum, but you will want to shoot for higher to look more appealing as an applicant. The good news is that if you don't do well, it's not the end of the world. You can always take the test again to try to get a better score. However, keep in mind that each time you take it, you have to pay the fee again, which is currently $205 as of the writing of this book.

Don't just take it on a whim. Study hard and schedule it when you know you're ready. You don't want to waste your time or money.

STEP 5

Get Letters of Recommendation

Most schools require at least 3 letters of recommendation. A good variety of people to get this from includes supervisors, co-workers, professors, and doctors. Don't simply get your friends to write good things about you. The admissions committee will be able to pick up on this right away.

During your time in the ICU, you should have been spending a good amount of time networking with all of these potential references. If you are the quiet nurse on the unit, it may be difficult finding someone who can give you a good recommendation.

Sometimes the recommendations can be written in free-form by the reference. But many times, the school will require a specific form to be filled out and a protocol to follow. They may have to seal the envelope and send it to the school themselves, so you may never get to see it. They do this to prevent any tampering with recommendations that didn't go the way you had hoped.

STEP 6
Observe a CRNA

Although I list this as one of the last steps, it probably also deserves a spot close to the top. It might be a good idea to see first-hand what a CRNA does before you go through all of this trouble. You may find out that it's not what you want to pursue after all. It's not for everyone, and the sooner you figure it out, the better.

Even if you do shadow someone in the beginning of your journey, you will also want to do it again before you apply to anesthesia school. This will help to confirm your decision to become a CRNA. Besides that, it is a requirement for admission at most programs.

Many schools will have the CRNA you are shadowing to sign a form stating that you were there. You might also have to write about your experience, as well as why you have decided to enter the profession.

While you are shadowing, try to get as much information from the CRNA as you can without annoying them. See if they enjoy what they do and why. Get a sense of how most of their days are spent—not just this particular one. How are their hours and do they have time for a life outside of work? This isn't really the time to learn about the technical aspects of anesthesia. Instead, just try to get an overall sense of what you will be doing if you're accepted into the school.

STEP 7
Apply to CRNA School

After completing all of the prerequisites, start applying. Admissions to CRNA school are unbelievably competitive, so it would be a good idea to apply to more than one. You will either be rejected immediately or invited for an interview for further consideration. If you don't get in, take a deep breath. Have a good cry, but then relax and go back to the drawing board. Instead of giving up, try again, and try again, and try again. Consider retaking the GRE to get a higher score, retaking old classes that you got poor grades in, or applying to different schools.

Consider applying to schools that are out of your area. In my class, over 20% of the students were from a different state. If becoming a CRNA is something you are determined to do, then you will have to make some sacrifices. Moving to a different place is tough, especially if you have a family. But it is short term. Once you graduate, you can live pretty much anywhere you want.

STEP 8
Nail the Interview

If you're lucky enough to get an interview, congratulations! The process of getting into CRNA school involves several 'weeding-out' processes. If you've made it to the interview stage, then you've gotten past hundreds of other applicants who have already been weeded out.

The truth is that the interview may not have a huge bearing over whether or not you get in. Usually, they have their minds pretty much made up and just want to see who they are opening the door to. With that said, it can make a difference if they are sort of on the fence and can't decide between you and another candidate. Also, they can sometimes tell how well you will do in their program based on your personality. Even if all of your qualifications are perfect, they still might not accept you if you totally bomb the interview.

Make sure you get there on time—and by 'on time,' I mean early. You don't want their first impression of you to be an interruption as you walk through the door late.

Dress professionally and try to relax. Now is not the time to skimp on your wardrobe. You may be able to get by with business casual, but I would just play it safe and dress in full business attire. You're not interviewing for McDonald's here.

They will likely first talk to all of the candidates as a group before they bring you in individually. Some schools may have you take a short aptitude test, just to see where your current knowledge base lies. If they give you this test, it doesn't mean wrong answers will get your application denied. They just want to know what you know.

When they speak to you one-on-one, try to stay calm. I know you will be nervous, but you must be able to think clearly. They aren't going to ask you tough questions. The idea is just to get to know you to see how well you'll fit into their program.

It's an interview for you to decide if they are right for you also. Just because they might accept you doesn't mean you have to go there.

Maybe the schedule isn't at all what you expected. Maybe the costs are out of your range. It could be anything. When they are done asking you questions, there will be time for you to ask some of them. Try to get some answers and don't be intimidated.

Lastly, just try to be yourself. If you're a good nurse and a good person, then you shouldn't have a problem. If it's meant to be, you'll get in!

PART 2

SURVIVE
CRNA SCHOOL

INTRODUCTION

Your story might be similar to mine, or maybe you always knew that becoming a CRNA is what you wanted. Anesthesia school is almost guaranteed to be more difficult than you expect. You'll begin to understand what I mean when you are waist deep in textbooks, trying to keep your eyes open to study after your 9th day in a row of clinicals. The goal of this book is not to teach you anesthesia. You will get much more than you bargained for in your respective CRNA School.

I'm not going to attempt to squeeze hundreds of texts, studies, and experiences into one short book. Instead, I will try to teach you some tips and tricks that might help you along the way, including how to deal with some of the emotional issues that might arise, how to study smarter, and how to interact with others in your field. I want you to be able to not only survive, but also thrive, over the next 2-3 years. Hopefully by the end of this book, you'll feel more prepared and confident to face the many challenges that are up ahead.

I decided to write this because I wish someone had shown me the ropes when I was a student. The scariest part of anything is the unknown, and I think you might all classify anesthesia school in the realm of the unknown. While this book won't be able to tell you exactly what to expect, it will hopefully alleviate some of the concerns you have and answer some burning questions for you. Take the advice if you think it will help, or simply ignore it if you think I'm full of it.

I know I don't have all the answers, but this is some of what I've learned in school and beyond. Feel free to skip around through the book as you please. I tried to separate it into sections that you can access quickly if you're just looking for specific information. If there is something you have a question about or would like further clarification on, please email me at contact@kickassnursing.com. If I left something out that you would like my opinion on, I would be happy to help as much as I can. I'm open to critique and suggestions for improvement, or you can just contact me to let me know how much the book sucks if you want.

CHAPTER ONE

You're In! Now You Can Relax (Well, if You Have Some Xanax)

You finally did it! After years of hard work and preparation, you've managed to beat out many of your peers to claim one of the few seats available in CRNA School. So pat yourself on the back, because just getting a foot in the door is a huge hurdle to jump. But after you breathe that sigh of relief, get ready to put in some hard work. The attrition rate for student nurse anesthetists can reach upwards of 10%, or more for some programs.

Not only am I going to teach you the things I learned when I was in CRNA School, but also some of the things I wish I would have learned. These strategies are not meant as a replacement for hard work and persistence. But hopefully they will help make things a little easier as you go through the long, difficult journey that lies ahead.

If you've made it to this point in your life, you've likely spent at least a couple of years in the

ICU or ER as a registered nurse. You are the cream of the crop in your unit and are well respected by all of your peers. Many of you may have been charge nurses, supervisors, or administrators. Your new reality as a student may be a difficult one to accept, and it will definitely take some time getting used to being the low person on the totem pole. The sooner you're able to accept it however, the sooner you'll be able to move on to succeeding in anesthesia school. You are now on equal footing with all of your classmates, most of you coming from similar situations. All the respect you've earned over your successful career vanishes instantly the first time you walk into that classroom. That's not to say that you won't regain that respect, but you will be starting from scratch.

Keeping that in mind, never forget where you came from. Just the fact that you're in CRNA School shows what you've accomplished so far in your career. Thousands of applications are submitted to nurse anesthesia programs throughout the country, while only a fraction of them are accepted. So even though you are on the low end of the totem pole, it is a pretty strong totem pole that plenty of people would love to be a part of.

There will be days that go by that test your patience and make you wonder why the heck you ever decided to put yourself through this. At times, you will feel incredibly small and may even want to cry. Stay grounded, but remember that you are a great nurse no matter what happens. No professor, preceptor, or anesthesiologist can take that away from you.

The first day of class may be a little overwhelming. You will be meeting the only people who can comprehend exactly what you are going through over the next 2-3 years. Everyone will be nervous, but try to make a good impression. Don't be a recluse like I was. Instead, make as many friends as you can as fast as possible. They can mean the small difference between becoming a CRNA and going back to the ICU. This is also a time when you meet some of your teachers, get your syllabus, and gain a general understanding of what's to come. Listen closely to the requirements and expectations for each class. Some important information might be given that isn't on the syllabus, so be sure to bring something to write with.

You will also be given a list of books, some of which are required and some which are simply suggestions. I would recommend getting every book on the list, and then find some more. You can never get enough information, and there is plenty out there. Some books will have conflicting data and different opinions. It's good to have a wide variety of resources so you can get the best information available.

Anesthesia is constantly changing, just like every other discipline in healthcare. Because of this, textbooks alone will not be able to keep up with these changes. Recent articles and studies can be a great resource for the latest information. You should always try to keep up with the latest trends in anesthesia. Not only will they advance your knowledge base, they also give you good conversation starters with your preceptors.

Although studies and articles are great for clinical development, almost everything you get graded on in class will come from materials presented in the syllabus. Time is a very valuable asset in CRNA School, so try to focus on the task at hand. It's great to keep up on the latest in anesthesia, but don't skip required reading to get it done. So, if you are getting tested on material from Basics of Anesthesia, then the article about flow-volume loops can probably wait. If you have an exam tomorrow on antibiotics in Pharmacology, don't start reading the latest studies on ischemic optic neuropathy in the prone position. Flow-volume loops and blindness during a spinal fusion are great topics to learn about, but the information can be absorbed another day.

CHAPTER TWO
Getting Your Textbooks

I'm sure I don't need to tell you how expensive textbooks can be. You probably have plenty of experience with this in your pursuit of a nursing degree. If you can afford it, just go ahead and get the books from the school bookstore. This will save you a lot of time and trouble in the long run, as it will ensure that you get the right book by the right author in the right edition. But as an SRNA without an income, you'll probably find it very important to make every penny count. No one would blame you if you decided to go another route. There are a few different options if you have to cut down on expenses in this area.

The first is to find them used on various web sites, such as eBay or Amazon. This has become very popular over the past few years, so there are several places to choose from. Some sites even act as a sort of liaison. For instance, at www.bigwords.com, you put the book information in the toolbar and it shows you all of the prices from various competitors. Shop around until you find the best deals. Just be careful, as some prices might be too good to be true. A really cheap textbook may have flaws, such as missing or ripped pages, lots of markings, etc. A book with a lot of writing and underlining in it may not seem like a big deal, but something like that can be very distracting when you are trying to focus on a specific topic.

You might also be able to buy some books very cheaply from upperclassmen or graduates of the program. Most students are running on empty towards the end of the program and right after graduation. They are looking for just about any way to make some extra money until they get that first paycheck. But again, if you go down this road, make sure the books are in the correct edition. Some of the textbooks are used again every semester, but they are often updated or changed entirely.

You could also rent your textbooks from sites like Chegg or Amazon. Make sure you search for your books by the ISBN number so you can make sure you have the correct one. I accidentally rented the British version of a textbook once in nursing school, and it made for a very difficult semester. Also, keep in mind that textbooks are usually rented by the semester. After the semester is over, you are required to send them back. I had to do this many times as I was running low on cash throughout the program. Later in the year, there was nothing I could do if I wanted to look back at something in the book. It would have been much more helpful for me to have all of my books when it came time to study for my comprehensive exams and boards.

The last option and one I would highly recommend against is that of sharing with your fellow classmates. It might seem like a good idea at first, but it will be a huge inconvenience as your program moves along. Unless you have the same schedules and always want to look at the same things, sharing will not be an easy task. You would have to sit next to each other in class with the book between the two of you, and you wouldn't be able to study exactly what you want whenever you wanted to. Anesthesia school is tough enough without having to worry about these types of silly things. It's just not worth the hassle to be able to save a little money. In short, whether they are new or used, buy your textbooks if you can. It will save you a huge headache in the long run.

CHAPTER THREE
Finding a Way to Pay for it

Paying for school is probably something you've already gotten a handle on if you've come this far. However, I think it's a subject that deserves some attention. I wasn't sure how I was going to finance everything until just before school started. I just focused mainly on getting into school, and I decided to worry about the money later. Financing can become a huge issue in CRNA School because there are very few, if any, programs that allow you to work while in school. So not only do you need to find a way to pay for tuition and books, but you also have to think about basic living expenses and lost wages for 2-3 years.

The most obvious way to pay for all of this is through student loans. Graduate students are eligible for up to $20,500 per year in unsubsidized Direct Loans. Any additional amount, up to the cost of attendance, can be achieved by taking out government PLUS loans for a slightly higher interest rate. Cost of attendance includes tuition, books, and living expenses. However, the financial aid office of the specific school you are attending determines the cost of attendance, not the government. So this amount may vary for each student from school to school. Even with all of this assistance, sometimes it's still not enough. This is especially true if you are a single parent or someone with a spouse who stays at home.

There is also the option of private student loans, which are much harder to come by these days. They are difficult to find, but some are available if you have decent credit. You might run across the same problem as government loans in that they will often cover only up to the cost of attendance. I had to rely on these a lot more than I wanted to, and I am paying for it now. Do what you have to do if it comes down to it, but try to stay away from these higher interest loans.

Another way to get some financial assistance is by applying for those elusive scholarships. These are extremely difficult to find and you typically have to be an academic star to get these. But there are some that just about anyone can get. You might have to write something on a specific subject, put in a certain amount of volunteer hours, or complete some sort of research. Your school's financial aid office should be able to help you find some of these opportunities. You may also be able to find some at the AANA (American Association of Nurse Anesthetists) web site or your state's Anesthesia Association. But don't stop there. There are several scholarships available for any Master's level degree, not just nurse anesthesia. Type in "master's scholarships" into any search engine and you'll see what I mean. With great persistence, I suppose it would be possible to find enough scholarship money to cover much of your tuition.

If you don't mind putting in some time for your country after graduation, you can get great financial help from the Army or Navy. In exchange for work after graduation, they will pay a monthly stipend to help cover your living expenses. The Army STRAP program now pays close to $2000 per month. They also offer student loan repayment to go along with this (up to $50,000 for reserves and $120,000 for active duty). It's a truly great thing to be able to give service to your country, but not everyone is cut out for it. Make sure this is something you are willing to commit to, as there is no going back once you sign. They will accept service in the form of active duty or reserves as a nurse anesthetist.

If the military isn't your thing, you could always look for anesthesia groups to pay for your tuition or give you a stipend each month. These are not easy to find, but there are still some out there. They will obviously want a commitment of some sort, so make sure you know what you are signing. You can call or email different groups to see if they would be interested in such an arrangement. The only catch is that they are usually looking for someone who has at least a year of anesthesia school under their belt. They also want someone who has decent grades and good clinical evaluations. Start your search at your own clinical sites. They already know your clinical skill and work ethic, and will be much more likely to work with you. Plus, it will be an easy transition when you graduate, going from an SRNA to a CRNA in the same place. Some people prefer to go somewhere different than their school's clinical site, fearing that they would be forever branded a "student" in the eyes of the anesthesiologists and other co-workers. When I graduated, I decided to stay at the same site, and I didn't find this to be an issue.

CHAPTER FOUR
Study Smarter, Not Harder

You know the old saying, "you can't pick your parents?" Well the same holds true for your teachers. You are going to have some teachers that you love, while there will be others who you could easily do without. Unfortunately, these aren't undergraduate courses that you can simply withdraw from. Ah, how I longed for those days in undergrad when we had a drop/add week in the beginning of the semester. If you didn't like a class for any reason, you could simply drop it and add a different one. Well this isn't undergrad, so you're pretty much out of luck if you're not happy. Instead of lamenting this fact, try to make the most of every class and every teaching style.

Talk to your upperclassmen so you know what's coming. You don't want any surprises. You may be able to listen to certain teachers and everything will click as the words flow from their mouths. There will likely be others whose lectures you have to record and listen to over and over. Learn their teaching styles, but more importantly, learn their testing styles. Find out if they go strictly from their lectures and power points, or if random items from the textbook also show up on exams. Previous students should be able to help you some with this information, but it may take a test or two to figure out what they're looking for.

In the beginning, try to cover all your bases. For instance, if there is a reading assignment on the schedule, make sure you read it. Don't just look at the notes from the lecture and the PowerPoint. It is a lot of work at first, but you will find it easier to manage your time as each class progresses. Most professors will give you some idea of their expectations at the start of each semester. But you'll find that most will show certain tendencies on their exams. While you should always study everything that's on the syllabus, you will want to focus more of your energy covering these tendencies.

It is vitally important for you to find a way to study that works for you. It's going to be impossible to learn everything that is thrown at you in CRNA School. Are you an audio, visual, or kinesthetic type of learner? Unless you have a photographic memory, it would be helpful to determine whether you learn best by listening to a lecture, looking at pictures and video, or by physically doing something. Many people already know what kind of learner they are, but there are lots of tests out there to find out if you're not sure. As classes move along, you will be able to hone in on the things that help you recall all of the information given to you.

When I was in school, almost all of the lectures were video recorded along with the PowerPoint presentation the professors worked from. So we could essentially go back and re-take the lecture as often as we would like. Whether your school does this or not, I would highly recommend recording the audio from the lectures yourself. This way, you will always have the file to reference back to at any time.

Many of my classmates would listen to these lectures whenever they were driving to and from class or clinicals. I tried this at first, but it never worked for me like it did for others. I would just find myself spacing out, thinking of much more interesting things while I drove. I ended up using that time to decompress a little, just listening to music or sports, trying not to think too much. Clearly I needed more than just audio recordings to get me through.

In my school, every lecture was presented by way of PowerPoint. I personally found it very difficult to study directly from these PowerPoints. Instead, I converted them all to a Microsoft Word document, allowing the words to flow more like a story instead of window after window. I am not very tech savvy, so I had to go through slide after slide, copying a pasting each paragraph. Then I would manually re-format every sentence and picture.

There must be an easier way to get this done, as it was very time consuming. If I had a few extra hours, I would sometimes transcribe the audio lecture into a word document also. This was usually a strategy reserved for those teachers that tested a lot of content from the lecture itself, information often left out of the PowerPoint or textbook itself. This was helpful during my first couple semesters, but became too difficult as I progressed in the program.

Something else that might work for you is to make questions and answers for the material. I used to go through every sentence of the

PowerPoints, formulating a question and answer for each. They can be simple true/false questions, multiple choice, or direct answer. Just this process alone accounted for most of my absorption of the material. The work isn't just mindless formatting. You have to think of a way to arrange a question that would be fitting for the answer. Working through each question this way was one of the best studying techniques I utilized during the program.

After I completed this, I would then take the questions and make flashcards out of them. You can make physical flashcards or create them online. There are also several apps that offer this function. Keep looking repetitively at 5-10 flash cards at a time, until you have them memorized, then move to the next. The idea is to work your way up to memorizing the entire stack.

These are great strategies, but many of them take up a lot of very valuable time, something which comes at a premium the further you move along in your program. Dividing the work will help immensely in saving you that precious time and energy. A good tip is to form a small group and have each person take turns transcribing audio, converting to Word, or making flashcards. You can set up a group web site for the entire class if you'd like, so everyone can post the things they've worked on. A couple of great sites for this are Quizlet and Dropbox. You could also get someone else to do some of the work for you. If you have the money, there are plenty of web sites that have freelancers who would love to transcribe audio or convert PowerPoints for a fee.

Mnemonics were also a huge help for me as I went through anesthesia school. There are several that are fairly well known, but you can make up just about anything that will help you remember. They don't even have to make sense, as long as they help you recall information better. For example, you might know one of the common mnemonics used to help you remember a basic set-up before any case. SOAPME was very useful during my first few months to help remember what I needed before starting any case. It stands for Suction, Oxygen, Airways (ET tube, LMA, etc), Positioning (proper padding, pillows, etc), Monitors/Meds, and Equipment. This is just one example of the hundreds I used while in school. Search for some on the internet or make some up on your own. It may seem silly, but they are a savior for many.

When it comes to studying, learn by trial and error. Repeat the techniques you used that helped you pass an exam, but discard the techniques that were a waste of time. You want to study smarter, not harder. You may not benefit from making flashcards or listening to recordings, but it would be a good idea to a least give it a try. When I was in school, I found myself grasping at anything that might give me some sort of advantage. If you find that you are acing your tests, then stick with whatever works. But if you think you could use a little help, try out some of the methods I mentioned.

CHAPTER FIVE
The Classmate Advantage

When I was in school, I played sort of the loner role. At least I believe that's how my classmates saw me. I am married with 3 kids, and I value my time with them very much. Between classes and clinicals, I barely saw them as it was. Because of this, I ended up arriving to class right before it started, and I would leave as soon as it was over. Most of my classmates would hang around the classroom to chat or meet up somewhere to study. While they were quizzing each other for the pharmacology exam, I was quizzing my son for his geometry exam. I always studied alone, usually after everyone else in my house had already gone to sleep.

Although I wouldn't change the way I approached it, I know that it caused me to skate a lot closer to the edge than many of my peers. I would strongly suggest that you make friends with as many of your classmates as possible. Form study groups and bounce ideas off each other. When you might be confused with a subject, they might say just the right thing to help it all sink in. Also, I believe that all of the study methods mentioned before will likely stick in your mind the more your talk about them with other people. Besides that, studying alone is not a whole lot of fun. You can find yourself spinning, reading passages over and over, realizing each time you have no idea what you just read. Having someone else there to snap you out of it makes a huge difference when it comes time for the test.

In your class, there are going to be a few students at the top and a few at the bottom. But most of you will find yourselves somewhere in between. If you don't understand something, ask your classmate. They will either know the answer already, or they are having the same trouble and you can figure it out together. Just make sure you're always there when another classmate needs helps from you. This symbiotic relationship also works well in clinicals.

Talk to each other about your experiences. Share your successes, share your failures, and then share your failures again. It's great to hear how fantastic one of your classmates did in their first intubation attempt, and that information may help you a little. They can tell you about their technique and walk you through the steps. But it's even more valuable information to hear about the intubation they missed. Find out what happened, why it happened, and what they could have done differently.

You can't succeed in anything until you fail a little. Try to learn from other people's errors as much as you can. But don't think that you will avoid all mistakes. You are going to make a few (ok, you are going to make a lot of) mistakes. But that's all part of becoming a great CRNA. As long as you learn from your past and avoid those same mistakes in the future, then you won't have any problems.

The CRNA's and anesthesiologists you work with were in your shoes at one time. They understand that you are there to learn, and most are very forgiving. When you slip up, acknowledge it, talk about it with your preceptor, and grow from it. You will gain much more from a bad day than you ever will from a good day. Don't forget to broadcast your mistakes to the rest of your classmates. They will appreciate it, just like you will when they tell you their stories.

Another great way to connect with your peers is by attending workshops and meetings offered by the AANA or your state's organization. These are excellent opportunities to meet other students and CRNAs from around the country. Often, your school will pay for you to attend or will reimburse you. I wish I had attended more of these when I was a student. They give you the chance to see what things are like in anesthesia in places outside of your clinical site. We often get used to things in our little bubbles, but if you dare to venture out you will find that there are many more ways of doing things. Also, you can get an amazing amount of training with the latest products in anesthesia. There are workshops available for difficult airway, regional anesthesia, and learning the business side of anesthesia. These are just a few options out there. During your time as an SRNA, try to keep track of when these things are offered and check with your school to see if it is something they'd be willing to foot the bill for.

CHAPTER SIX
Setting Up Before Cases

At the beginning of each day, I always start with my machine check. The newer machines require little more than pressing a few buttons, but you really should learn how to do a traditional check on an older machine. Once the machine is checked, make sure you have working suction. Many would suggest that this is the first thing you should always do, and maybe it is. The reason I do the machine check first is to get the process started. Since the newer machines have self-checks that take a few minutes, I do everything else while it's cooking. As long as the suction gets checked before you start a case, I'm not sure it matters when you do it.

Next, I make sure there is adequate oxygen supply in the tank, just in case the wall supply malfunctions. I've never had to use it, but you never know.

Then I make sure I have a working ambu bag and mask. Get your tape ready for the eyes and have the tape ready to secure the ET Tube once it's in place. The order you do these things doesn't matter as much as making sure they all get done. It's important to have a routine in place, doing the same steps in the same order every time. If you do this, it's much less likely that you'll forget something.

Once everything is checked, I always make an emergency set-up in addition to each specific case. I get a couple of different sized ET Tubes prepared, along with a variety of oral airways. I keep them covered and usually don't have to use them. But I always have them ready. Aside from emergencies, they may also come in handy if your tube accidentally gets dropped during intubation (as you can imagine, it's not really a good idea to pick up a tube from the ground and stick it into someone's trachea). Unfortunately, this has actually happened on occasion (not to me, of course!). But it wasn't a big deal because the backup tubes were already waiting in the wings. Trust me...the day you don't have them ready is the day you'll wish you had. I'm sure some of you remember being in the ICU with a patient you just didn't feel right about. You would bring the code cart in front of the room to ward off evil spirits.

Well, it's the same idea for your emergency set-up.

After I have my back up supplies prepared and everything checked, I start setting up for the specific case I expect to be managing. For a general anesthesia case requiring intubation, I first make sure to put out the ET Tube. In my facility, we typically use a 7.0 ET Tube for a female and a 7.5 ET Tube for a male. If the patient is expected to stay intubated after the case, we will usually use an 8.0. The preference of the ET Tube size varies from site to site, so make sure you know the typical sizes used in your facility.

When setting up an ET Tube, first push the plastic connector into the tube itself to make sure it is snug. Put the stylet into the tube and bend it to preference. I personally prefer a hockey stick appearance with a small curve at the end. Make sure the stylet is not past the murphy's eye at the end of the tube. You can bend the top of the stylet near the connector to make sure it can't slip further down. Next, take a 10 cc syringe and test the pilot balloon to make sure there are no leaks. After this meets your satisfaction, withdraw all of the air back into the syringe.

Next to the ET tube, have your intubating blade of preference. I like to keep both of them out and next to each other. This way, if I am unsuccessful with one type of blade, I could make a second attempt with the other. Your anesthesiologist might prefer a different blade than you do also. You never know if they will have to intubate after your attempts. Near the tube and the blades, have an oral airway, a tongue depressor, and a soft bite block (made from rolled 4x4 gauze). Have something ready to monitor the patient's temperature. The esophageal probe is preferred, but you can also monitor with a nasopharyngeal probe, or skin probe. You might get lucky if the patient has a Foley catheter in with a temperature probe attached. Also, have a couple of ekg pads to monitor twitches during paralysis.

For a general anesthesia case that calls for an LMA, the setup is a little different. Remember, no matter what type of anesthesia you're doing, you should always be prepared to intubate. Fortunately, this preparation was already done with your back up/emergency pack. Typical LMA sizes are 3 for a female, 4 for a male (or larger female), and 5 for a large male. You will see the typical suggested weight for each LMA size on the packaging. This is just a guide, and usually you can't determine an accurate size until you look at the patient. Lightly lubricate the outside of the cuff (not the part that will be facing the airway) and take out a few cc's of air. The amount of air you should take out is purely subjective. Some people take out all of the air, while others don't take any out. I think most CRNAs are somewhere in the middle, taking out just a little. Next to your LMA, have your oral airway, soft bite block, and tongue depressor. Just remember that an LMA will not protect against aspiration! You will be reminded of this approximately 500,000 times throughout your time as an SRNA, so don't forget it!

For a MAC (Monitored Anesthesia Care) case, you need to make sure you have a nasal cannula that will also monitor etCO2. These types of cases require a great deal of vigilance, as you have no airway protection. The patient is breathing on their own without an airway device, and your goal is to keep it this way. Have oral airways close by and have your suction even closer. As always, make sure you have an ET Tube and blade at the ready in case things go bad. It is never *just* a MAC, though you will hear this said many times. It generally takes a lot more skill to manage these types of cases than one in which an advanced airway is already in place.

Certain medications are drawn up for each specific case, but there are some standard things you will always want to have ready. First of all, succinylcholine is your friend. Keep it ready just in case. It can get you out of a jam in a hurry. You will also want to have some vasopressors ready in case of hypotension. Phenylephrine and Ephedrine are good choices, and the first ones most facilities use. Gylcopyrrolate is another great drug that should be ready to go in case of bradycardia. In my facility, these drugs are usually prepared ahead of time by the pharmacy. However, you will have to mix your own in some places.

For starters, know how to mix Ephedrine and Phenylephrine. If Ephedrine is in the usual 50 mg/mL vial, then you would take 1 mL and add it to 9 mL of saline to result in a push concentration of 5 mg/mL. Phenylephrine is usually in a 10 mg/mL vial. Take 0.1 mL (1 mg) and add it to 9.9 mL of saline to reach a push concentration of 100 mcg/mL. Keep in mind that different facilities might use different concentrations. Of course, as always, make sure the typical emergency drugs, such as epinephrine and Atropine, are ready and available should the need present itself.

There are 2 blades most commonly used for intubation. These would be the curved Macintosh (Mac) and the straight Miller blade. A Mac is used to slide to the back of the tongue into the vallecula, which will lift the epiglottis indirectly to hopefully reveal a beautiful grade I view of the vocal cords. Conversely, the Miller blade is inserted under the epiglottis, lifting it directly to get the view you're looking for. It's really a matter of preference as to which blade you should use.

It is typically a good idea to start out with the Mac as a student. It is more helpful in identifying anatomy and usually comes easier to most. Once you have done several intubations, you can start using the Miller more and more often. Most people will develop a favorite blade, but try to become proficient with both. While I can use the Miller if I need to, I feel more comfortable using the Mac blade. However, you will notice that many experienced clinicians will use the Miller almost exclusively.

CHAPTER SEVEN
Big Pimpin' (Working With Preceptors)

Preceptors will often quiz you during your time in clinicals with them. Sometimes the questions will be related to the case, while other times the questions are pulled from left field. This quizzing is commonly known in many SRNA circles as getting "pimped." Some of your preceptors are asking you these questions because they genuinely want to help advance your learning. Other preceptors are honestly just trying to figure out how far along your knowledge base is. Finally, there are some preceptors who simply get a kick out of watching you squirm. I think some of it has become the culture to give students a hard time. Many CRNAs weren't treated with kid gloves when they were in school either, and they view it as a rite of passage. I think a little tough love is necessary sometimes if it helps you grow as an anesthesia provider. But I don't think being mean for the sake of being mean is the right way to go about it.

I know it's going to be difficult, but please try not to think of getting pimped in a negative way. Believe it or not, the questions I remember most vividly from school didn't come from any lecture or exam. They came during intubations, line placements, and titrating of anesthesia. It can sometimes be very hard to stumble through question after question when you are struggling to just get the tube through the cords. But those questions and discussions during cases are the ones that will likely be forever burned in your memory. With that said, it would look much better for you to get a majority of these questions correct.

Make sure you know your stuff, especially the basics. You absolutely have to have your top drawer meds memorized. This means dosing, onset, duration, method of action, and indications. If you've known in advance which case you are doing, you should know all of the anesthetic implications. You should know what to expect in the case, how much blood is lost on average, and things that you might need to do differently in comparison with other cases.

Try to look up your patient's information well in advance of the case. This way, you can research their specific disease processes and know how it will impact the care you give them. You can look up their medications and determine if any of them affect your anesthetic plan also. It will be seen as inexcusable in many preceptors' eyes to miss those sorts of things if you've had time in advance to look everything up. Of course there will be many times when you get a new case that you haven't had time to research. Your preceptor will be more understanding in this scenario, but you will need to learn to adapt to change and know how to find information on the fly.

If you don't know the answer to a question, try to start with something you do know that's related and work your way through it in your head. If you absolutely don't know something, then say so. But let your preceptor know that you will get back to them with an answer. Make sure you follow up on this! That night, research the topic and write about your findings. They are not expecting a novel here, but it should be more than a couple sentences. Make it look like you cared about what they were asking you. A couple paragraphs should suffice for most things. Try to find that preceptor the next morning to hand it to them or put it in their box. If they have time, see if they will discuss it with you.

I would strongly suggest that you keep a file of questions you have been asked along with the answers. Our class kept a file titled "pimp questions" that could be accessed by all of the students. So if I knew I was going to be with a specific preceptor, I could look in that file to see what types of questions had been asked before by them.

On days you are with a preceptor, try to make a good impression. It goes beyond a flawless intubation and seamless wake up. No matter how well you do technically, it won't mean anything if you are difficult to work with. It's ok to be a little quiet. Sometimes that is preferred over some of the alternatives. However, try to be personable. When they aren't asking you questions, try to think of something good to ask them, or follow up on something they've already talked about. It will make you seem interested and involved in the case, which is much better than being disengaged. Make sure the questions you ask don't have obvious answers that you should already know. You may end up shooting yourself in the foot.

I would recommend that you don't ask the same question twice, even if it's directed to a different preceptor. It shows a definite lack of interest. Either you didn't care enough to remember what the answer was, or you were only asking because you wanted to *seem* interested. It may not be that big of a deal to most, but why take the chance?

While we're on the subject, try to ask questions that will help you get better. Ask things like "do you have any pointers or tips to improve my intubation technique?" You might also ask something like "what are some of the different ways this could be done?" The point here is to make sure your preceptor knows that you aren't just there simply because you're on the schedule. Show them that you are interested and want to learn, and most will be more than happy to teach you.

It would also be a very good idea to have a general preceptor preferences file. You will quickly find out that every CRNA and anesthesiologist has a different way of doing things. Keep a detailed file on your computer of every preceptor you've been with. Remembering little things that each person does differently will go a long way. Although you might be with a new preceptor every day, they might only have a student once or twice a week. They are likely to remember the things they told you and the things you've discussed together.

Keep track of things such as where certain people like to keep their eye tape before induction: on the mask, on the machine, or somewhere else? Do they like to use a specific gas more than most? What is their preferred method to get patients breathing? Do they like to use a lot of narcotics? You get the idea.

In the end, it shouldn't matter how you do things, as long as there is a valid reason and it works. But it definitely will matter to most of your preceptors until you are much further along and they have gained a certain level of comfort working with you. I have a specific routine that keeps my mind right, as will most other CRNAs you are with. Everything is in the same spot for every case. If I have to reach for something quickly, I know exactly where it is because it's always there. Although every case is unique, there is a basic way

I do my inductions, maintenance, and emergence. It's easy to get rattled if something is out of place or different in some way. So try not to get annoyed when your preceptor keeps redirecting you to do things their way.

As you move further along as an SRNA, you are going to learn to take the good things you see and hopefully leave the bad. You will eventually have your own way of doing things. But when you are first getting started, try to learn what they want and duplicate it the next time you are with them. Encourage your classmates to do the same so you can share information with each other.

CHAPTER EIGHT

*Maintaining Confidence
While Getting the Most
Out of Your Clinical Time*

Try to remember back to your first clinical day in nursing school. Most of you probably can still feel that very real urge to throw up. Well, your first day of clinicals in CRNA School will likely be much worse. At least it was for me. It took most of my first year before the butterflies in my stomach began to fade. This might not be a huge problem for some of you. But then again, I would frankly be concerned if you weren't the slight bit nervous. It shows that you're human and that you understand the seriousness of what you're getting yourself into. These patients are real and we hold their lives in our hands. Any mistakes or missteps can have disastrous consequences. This is something that you always need to remember no matter how far along you are in your career.

With that in mind, try to temper your nerves as much as possible. Even if you are scared as hell on the inside, show nothing but confidence on the outside. This will help tremendously to put your preceptors at ease, not to mention the patients and their families. It may sound strange, but the more they believe in you, the more you will believe in yourself. If your preceptors see the fear in your eyes, they will be more likely to look for flaws. They will probably ask you more questions to find out how much you really know. If you look like you know what you're doing, more often than not, they are happy to just let you do your thing.

Once you get over those initial butterflies and you've cleaned yourself up, try to stop running the other way when something unfamiliar presents itself. Use your time as a student CRNA wisely, and try to get as many experiences as possible. Don't be afraid of looking stupid, because now is the time to learn. It will look a lot worse if you don't know how to do something after you graduate.

Ask your preceptors and attending doctors if you can get as many opportunities as possible. Watch central line placements enough times and then ask if you can try doing some. If your patient is a difficult intubation, ask if you can get a look with the fiber optic scope. Ask to get your hands on things even when your patient isn't a difficult intubation. Healthy patients with easy airways are good ones to learn things like the lightwand, bougie, Glidescope, fiberoptic, etc. Practice now so you will know how to use these things when they are really needed. Ask your preceptor if you can try using different medications or anesthetic techniques that you don't have much experience with. If there is an interesting case, see if you can go help out or at least observe. You are only an SRNA once, so make the most of your time in school.

Don't worry about things like missing an intubation, having difficulty masking, difficulty putting in an a-line, etc. These are the things you will get better with every time you do it. While we're on the subject, I should clarify what I mean by "missed intubation." It can be defined in a few different ways. For example, you might struggle to get a good view, so you hand over the blade to your preceptor. If they are able to get a good view easily without doing much differently, I would consider that a miss. If you put the tube in the esophagus instead of the trachea, that's a clear miss. We would refer to that as "tubing the goose."

Don't get discouraged by these times. They happen to everyone, even experienced CRNAs from time to time. During intubation, make sure you tell your preceptor or attending exactly what you see as you go. If you don't have a great view, let them know. Don't intubate blindly unless you are instructed to. If your preceptor thinks you have a good view, it is not going to go well if you tube the goose. On the other hand, if your preceptor allows you to try to intubate with a difficult view, then it won't look nearly as bad.

You are also going to have difficulty masking certain patients. I haven't met anyone that was an expert at masking their first day, or even their first couple of years. It's one of the hardest things in anesthesia to get down. Have your oral airway ready, but try to master it as much as you can without one. Watch other people mask and try to learn from them. Be sure to put your fingers on the jawbone, not the soft tissue. Lift the jaw towards the mask, rather than pressing down on the face. Lift the mask as needed to let some trapped air out, creating your own sort of pop-off valve.

You're likely going to hear these same tips hundreds of times, but only because they will help you accomplish the lofty goal of achieving gas exchange in the lungs. Lastly, the only tried and true way to become very good at intubation and masking is by practice, over and over again. Failure isn't true failure when you're in anesthesia school. Sure, it hurts in the moment. But it's what makes you better in those same situations in the future.

CHAPTER NINE

Coming to Terms With Your New Hectic Schedule

I've heard many stories about CRNA students whose personal lives unravel a little while in school. It's hard to keep a relationship with your new busy schedule. Many end up breaking it off with girlfriends and boyfriends or getting divorced from their spouse. It's a sacrifice for your family as much as it is for you, if not even more so. When I started my anesthesia training, I was married with 2 small children. I'm happy to say that we stayed married through everything and even added a 3rd baby to the mix. But it was definitely a trying experience for all of us. My children had a hard time understanding why I had to stay late at the hospital, then come home and study all night. My wife knew what I was up against, but it still wasn't easy for her to accept some of our time apart.

Before you start school, have a long talk with your family. If you have children, be sure to include them in the discussion. Explain the specifics of what is required to get through the program. Make sure they understand that all of the time spent apart now is to prepare for a better future for all of you. On days before an exam, don't just go in your room or office and start studying. Spend a little time first telling them what you are doing and why. It will help, but it certainly won't fill that void you've left.

Lots of hard work and dedication are required to finish CRNA School, but you can't forget about the very people you're doing it for. Take a night off from studying here and there. Spend a weekend at the beach every once in a while. Make a date at the movies with your significant other. Hard work is necessary, but enjoy yourself also. Try to keep a good balance between school and home. It will make things easier for your family, and it will also help you keep your own sanity.

If you are single without children, it may be a little easier for you to deal with this aspect. But that isn't to say that it won't be hard also. In some ways, it may be a little more difficult without that close support system. Be sure to have someone to lean on when things get tough, because they certainly will. Make sure you always have someone to talk to, whether it be friends, family, or classmates.

Not only do you need to find a balance between school and home, but you also need to find a balance between the clinical and didactic portions of your program. I think one of my biggest mistakes when I first started CRNA School was that I focused an enormous amount of my attention on the clinical aspects, largely overlooking much of the didactic portion. I was so nervous about looking stupid during a case, I would spend most of my time reading about techniques or studying topics I thought I might get pimped on. As my grades began to sink, I knew I had to find a different strategy. It's important to find some kind of balance between clinicals and classes. If you do great on your exams and have a 4.0 gpa, it will mean nothing if you can't get through clinicals. On the other hand, if you are doing great in the hospital, it also won't matter if your grades are suffering.

Try to find your sweet spot. I would lean towards spending more study time on didactics, but you have to decide for yourself what needs the most work at which time. I think that if you spend the proper study time in your classes, the clinical knowledge will just come by itself. It's impossible to know what a preceptor might ask you, and studying everything all at once is futile. Clinical technique will come with practice and persistence. Plus, performance reviews are subjective and you will often get the benefit of the doubt if you show that you are trying. Exams are very much objective and can't be interpreted to mean anything other than pass or fail. This is just my opinion, but one I wish I would have had from the start. It would have made things go much easier for me.

When it comes to deciding when to show up for clinicals, a general rule of thumb is to make sure your preceptor doesn't beat you there. It is going to show that you are interested and ready to work if you are already in the room by the time they get there. It would be even better if you had your set up done and you were ready to discuss the case. This might not always be possible, as some CRNA's get to work pretty early. As long as you get there in plenty of time to set up, talk to the patient, and go over the anesthetic plan, you shouldn't have any problems.

When I first started CRNA School, I used to get to my clinical site at 5:30am for cases that didn't start until 7:30am. If that seems early, well...it's because it is. I wanted to make sure I had plenty of time to do everything I needed and study up if my case was unexpectedly changed. But I ended up spending a lot of time just sitting around after I had the room ready. As my program got further along, I started getting to the hospital at 6:00, 6:15, and eventually 6:30 in my last couple of semesters. The time you get there is completely up to you. Start out earlier than you think you need and see what works best. Usually no one will care what time you got there as long as you're ready to go.

While we are on the subject of working hours, we should discuss how you deal with the end of your shift also. Many programs will let you leave at the end of your scheduled shift, provided that there is someone else there to take care of the patient if you are still in a case. Sometimes, you might have to stay if there is no coverage. If you decide to stay and finish a case past your scheduled time on your own, this will be very much appreciated by your preceptor and the anesthesia gods will smile down upon you. However, I would recommend keeping this within reason. If the case should be finished within the next 30-60 minutes, then staying is probably the right choice. But if the case could go for another 5 hours, I don't think anyone would think less of you if you decided to leave. Use your own judgment and try to read your preceptor. Sometimes you can tell if they are expecting you to stay or if they don't care either way. If a preceptor insists on sending you home, don't fight it. If you really want to stay, ask politely if it would be ok if you finished the case. But if they keep telling you to go, then get the heck out of there.

CHAPTER TEN
Staying Off the Radar

As you go through anesthesia school, keep it a main goal of yours to stay out of the news, so to speak. Keep your head down and don't cause any waves. You don't want to be remembered for anything other than being a hard worker. Make sure they are aware that you know your stuff, but don't be a "know it all."

If you disagree with someone, ask politely if they can explain their reasoning. Present your case and ask what they think. But don't argue with anyone or flat out tell them they are wrong about something. Even if you know without a shadow of a doubt that you are right, just let it go. Talk about it with your teachers and classmates for verification and move on. Try to go with the flow.

Remember that you are a guest and you have to play ball their way. Try not to get caught up in the gossip. Instead, just keep your eye on the prize. Worry about yourself and no one else. The last thing I'd mention about this has to do with politics and religion. Just like they don't belong at the dinner table, they don't belong in the OR (at least not as far as you're concerned). We all know how passionate people can be, so it would behoove you to keep such opinions to yourself.

Don't burn any bridges while you're in school, as it's always better to keep your options open. If you decide that you'd like to work for the anesthesia group at your clinical site, then of course you want to make a good name for yourself. But even if you want to work somewhere else, your reputation may travel right along with you.

Many CRNAs and anesthesiologists know each other across the country. Just because you plan on living in another state doesn't mean your name won't follow you. Plus, someday you may want to come back. So don't get on anyone's bad side. Always keep your word and let them know you are there to do whatever is needed. Don't try to find the easy way out, always be available, and always look for new opportunities. Be honest and open and your good name will always stay with you no matter where you end up.

CHAPTER ELEVEN
Preparing for the Unexpected

As much as we would all like to prepare for our day before we go into the hospital, the cold hard truth is that we often have no idea what's coming our way until it's right in front of us. It's ok if you don't know the answer to something, as long as you know how to find the answers. Even as CRNA's, we often come across procedures or diseases that we haven't seen before. But we know where the resources are so we can be as informed as possible before a procedure starts.

I think it is of vital importance to have some kind of electronic device that you can quickly find information on. If you're like many people, you probably already have a smart phone. If you do, then there are plenty of apps and web sites that have tons of information that can be accessed quickly. If you don't have a smart phone, I would recommend getting one before you start clinicals. I don't go a day without looking up a medication, a dose, or condition. The alternative to this is to carry several books around with you, something which may not even be allowed in the OR at your facility.

While I won't recommend any specific apps for your phone, I can tell you the different kinds you should probably have. Be sure to have a drug guide of some sort, preferably one specific to anesthesia. You should be able to quickly find a medication's dose, onset, duration, method of action, and administration instructions. It should tell you how to mix and administer commonly used drips. You also need quick access to surgical procedures and anesthetic implications for each.

Another great help is to have a reference for specific disease states and how to manage them. I've seen some apps that cover each of the topics all in one place. Lastly, a simple search for things on the internet usually doesn't let me down. In fact, unless I'm looking up a drug, Google is usually my first stop to find information quickly. You can always ask another CRNA or anesthesiologist if you aren't familiar with something. I've been bailed out by my colleagues more times than I can count. Just remember, you don't necessarily have to know it all, but you have to know where to find it!

In the ICU or ER, you are usually surrounded by several other nurses who are there within seconds whenever an emergency arises. But in the operating room, you are in charge of dealing with emergencies until the anesthesiologist gets there. If your patient codes, you are the one calling the shots until then. It might take a few minutes for them to get there to take over, which is a long time when a patient isn't breathing or is in V-Fib.

You absolutely have to know your BLS, ACLS, and PALS. In CRNA only groups, you will be the last stop, so it becomes even more important. In the ICU, this is something that might be easily forgotten (at least the details) since you can rely so heavily on other people. I know I let some things slip away in the time between my re-certifications. But in the OR, you have to act quickly and decisively. Don't forget that there are many more types of emergencies than the dreaded code. You need to know what to do in case of malignant hyperthermia, airway fires, laryngospasm, and bronchospasm, among other things. Know where the meds are and know where the carts are. Don't be afraid to call for help and know what you need to do in the first few minutes before that help gets there.

The other piece of advice I can give you is to try not to freak out when something bad or unexpected happens. It's always been said that CRNAs are paid so well because we are able to handle such situations. We're not making six figures because we can intubate someone and put some gas on. It's because of our ability to respond quickly in emergencies and unpredictable circumstances.

As a CRNA, you must be able to adapt quickly. You can lose an airway or blood pressure in an instant. In one minute, you're waiting to roll back with your basic cystoscopy. In the next, that case is getting bumped for an emergency thoracotomy for a gunshot wound. You can prepare all day long, but anything can happen at any time. As Forrest Gump's momma would always say, anesthesia is like a box of chocolates...you never know what you're gonna get.

CHAPTER TWELVE
The Pre-op Interview and Post-op Report

Before surgery, you are going to interview every patient unless it is an emergent case. The goal is to find out as much useful information as possible to help guide your anesthetic plan. First introduce yourself and confirm the patient's identity. Check their allergies and NPO status. Then go over the patient's medical and surgical history. If it helps, start at the head and work your way down the body.

See if the patient or their family have ever had any complications related to anesthesia. Check their airway, looking at mallampati score, cervical range of motion, thyromental distance, neck size, and dentition. There may be a few more things your school or preceptor would also like for you to document in your airway examination. Make note of any missing, chipped, cracked, or loose teeth. Get a list of the patient's medications and make note of any anesthetic implications for each. As you do these exams more and more, it will get easier and faster. It may take you a while to go through each thing at first, but it will eventually become seamless and routine.

While you're in pre-op, make sure your patient has working IVs. If the case is complex or the patient has a cardiac history, an a-line may be required. If so, make sure it's in place before you go back to the operating room unless there is a reason to wait. Check all of the labs to make sure everything is normal or acceptable. If you think you might need blood during the case, make sure the patient is typed and crossed. Verify which antibiotics are ordered and know when they need to be re-dosed.

Lastly, make sure your patient understands what is going to happen to them and what to expect. I usually explain that we will go back to the operating room and will have them move over to another bed. I tell them that I will hook up the monitors, put an oxygen mask over their face, and then call in the anesthesiologist to come in to help them go to sleep. Make sure they know when they will be going to sleep. If not, many patients will start to get nervous as you enter the operating room and move over to the bed. You will likely hear them say, "You know I'm not asleep yet, right?" It's vital to set expectations for every patient. You might have done this a hundred times, but they haven't and are curious about what's going to happen and when.

Once a case is complete, you will take your patient to the recovery room or ICU, making sure you have oxygen and medications if needed while transporting. When giving report to the receiving nurse, try to be short and to the point. They aren't looking for the patient's biography here. Give a brief medical history, including allergies and pertinent medications. List the amount of fluid given, blood lost, blood given, and urine output. Tell them which antibiotics were given, as well as any narcotics.

You don't need to mention every anesthetic medication you administer. The nurse doesn't usually need to hear that you had the patient on Sevoflurane, that you gave 80mg of Lidocaine, or that you reversed the paralytic with Neostigmine and Robinul. They already assume you did all these things with most patients. Instead, just tell them the things you gave that were out of the ordinary. Of course, there will occasionally be a nurse that does want every detail and who asks a lot of questions. That is fine, but you typically don't need to waste your time giving this information. They usually don't want to hear it any more than you want to tell them.

Before you leave PACU, chart the vital signs and make sure the patient is stable. No one will fault you for spending a longer time in recovery to get them stabilized. If the patient's oxygen saturation is low, help the nurse get a nasal cannula, mask, or whatever is needed to fix the problem. If the blood pressure is too high or too low, then you need to get it back within an acceptable range before you leave.

If the patient is having pain, please try to help alleviate it as much as you can. Although the nurse will have orders for pain medication, they will appreciate it greatly if you don't leave someone screaming in agony as you walk away. After all, pain relief is a major part of what we do, and it looks poorly on our profession when we don't get the job done. While you should try to get to your next case quickly, it shouldn't come at the cost of your patient's safety or comfort.

CHAPTER THIRTEEN
Working With Others

You are going to be working with a lot more people than CRNAs and anesthesiologists. On a daily basis, you will be interacting with pre-op and PACU nurses, circulating nurses, surgical techs, anesthesia LPNs/techs, pharmacists...well you get the idea. These people can make your life much easier, but it will be more difficult for them if you don't get along. The best piece of advice I can give is to be nice! Make a good impression and try to be personable. Make sure you have a good attitude and be helpful when you can. You can't take care of any patient by yourself. You will need help getting supplies, positioning patients, getting meds, etc.

Of course, even if you're a jerk, you will still get the things you need. No one is going to sacrifice the well-being of a patient. But it might take a little longer to get non-emergency things, and they will likely not do it cheerfully. You will be able to feel the tension for sure. Anesthesia is hard enough. We need all the help we can get and we're happy to get it. I will say one more thing about Anesthesia LPNs/techs. If you are lucky enough to have them at your facility, treat them like gold. They are your lifeline, setting up in between cases, getting supplies, picking up meds, etc. I have not worked in a facility without them, and I can't imagine how much more stress that would cause.

Although it is important to be someone who is easy to get along with, you also don't want to be a pushover. Patient safety should always be your top priority. Don't let anyone rush you into making a poor decision. For example, there will be times when your patient will take a long time to wake up. There might be several people standing in the room waiting for you to extubate them so they can flip the room for the next case. The patient would probably be fine, but you just aren't quite comfortable yet. You will be tempted to pull the ET tube, thinking it's worth the gamble. Please don't do this. Don't do anything until you're ready. I'd rather have the turnover take a few minutes longer than the patient have to be re-intubated.

This doesn't just go for extubation of course. Don't ever start a case if you don't have everything you need to be safe. You might have those eyes on you again impatiently waiting. But do what you think is the safest thing. Also, don't ever let anyone move your patient without you taking care of the airway. Make sure everyone moves them on your count, with very few exceptions. These are just a few examples. You are going to experience many more of these types of issues every day. Just remember that patient safety is paramount. If you're not ready, then nothing should happen until you are.

CHAPTER FOURTEEN
Getting Certified and Finding a Job

When school first starts, I'm sure the last thing you'll be thinking about is your Board Exam. Frankly, I don't blame you. You can't walk before you crawl, and you really should take things one day at a time. But keep the end game in the back of your mind as you move along. In other careers and in other classes, it's ok to take a test and then forget everything you studied. In anesthesia school, this type of thinking will surely come back to bite you. There is a lot of information that you won't be able to cram in 2 weeks before your certification exam.

Try to think of every lecture, every class, and every case as job training rather than school. It makes it much easier to remember things knowing that the information will help you be better in your profession. You're not just studying for a test...you're studying for a career. Once you've gotten about a year of school under your belt, it would probably be a good time to start gradually spending more time getting ready for the final showdown. Think about signing up for a review course like the one offered by Valley Anesthesia. They offer several comprehensive weekend courses throughout the year around the United States. You can also try a program like Prodigy Anesthesia. They offer online exam simulation and tons of study material. Both of these options are pretty expensive, but they offer great preparation for boards and help tremendously with your confidence.

Unfortunately, I didn't have the funds for either of these programs. I was fortunate enough to get some old information from a previous student, but I procrastinated much longer than I should have. Although I passed the exam on the first try, I did not feel well prepared at all. I took the maximum amount of questions and I was sweating it out the entire way through. Don't do what I did. Focus mostly on your classes and your clinicals, but don't forget what is waiting at the end. Instead, make a plan and stick to it as much as you can. Try to answer 10 practice questions every day to start and go from there. If that proves to be too much, then make at least one day a week for it. Do what you can, but do it consistently. It will pay off in the long run!

It's hard to say at what point you should start looking for a job. Many employers won't hire you unless you're within 6 months of graduation. With that said, I'm sure there are several exceptions, particularly if you are looking to stay on at your current clinical site. The groups you have been working with know you pretty well after a fairly short period of time. Some may be willing to sign you during your first year. However, I think most students usually find a job in that final 6 months. For my program, we graduated in May. Almost all of my class had a position lined up by February.

Try not to wait until the last minute to decide where you want to work. It can be a fairly easy process to find a job, or it can be very difficult. It's not that you won't be able to find work. Rather, it's more likely that there will be an overwhelming amount of positions available. If you know you want to work in a specific area, then the job hunt will come much easier for you. However, if you are open and willing to move anywhere, then it might take some time deciding the best fit for you. There are many types of jobs for CRNAs out there. You could work at a major trauma center or a more rural hospital. You could get a job at a GI center, surgery center, or pain clinic. Whatever you decide, try not to sign into a contract longer than a couple of years. You don't want to be stuck somewhere if you're miserable.

If you do sign a contract, read it carefully. Even better, have a lawyer read it. If there is something you don't agree with, propose changes and have them send another contract to you. While you have a long time to decide where you want to work, keep in mind that there is a credentialing process that a CRNA must go through for any place they want to work. This can sometimes take 3-4 months to get finalized before you can begin working. The sooner they can get started on it, the sooner you can start your career. Make sure you have enough money in the bank to cover that time without a paycheck or student loans.

Start your job search at one of the many sites offering this service specifically for anesthesia providers. Create a profile and build you resume. Include information that is related to the position of nurse anesthesia. Most employers won't care that you worked at a coffee shop for 3 years after high school. Be sure to document where you went to nursing school and where you worked as a registered nurse. Because nurse anesthesia is a profession in such high demand, many employers likely won't give your resume much thought. Just make it look professional, so they know you are someone who can be taken seriously. As long you passed an accredited CRNA program and got certified, they are usually more than happy to have you as an employee. Your grade point average and the quality of your papers probably won't even be considered. Keep this in mind as you go through your program and receive a grade less than you hoped for. In the end, everyone who makes it all the way through will be given the title of CRNA.

After you graduate, make sure you take a break before you begin working. You are going to deserve some time to yourself to decompress. Try to go on vacation if you can. Either go before you take your board exam or wait until you've passed it to celebrate. I was dead broke when I graduated, so I just stayed at home. But I took the first week after school to just relax and spend time with my family. Then I hit the books hard and didn't stop until the exam. On the day of the exam, you should find out right after you submit your final answer whether or not you passed. Once you have that paper in your hand, feel free to tell the world how awesome you are...you've earned it!

CHAPTER FIFTEEN
Don't Stop Believing

I would love to tell you that reading this book is a guarantee of success, but the fact is that some people just aren't cut out for anesthesia. The same holds true for almost any profession. Sometimes all the determination in the world isn't enough to make a CRNA. It doesn't mean that the intelligence isn't there. It just means that they are meant to do something different.

Some people find this out during the first or second semester on their own, so they decide to go back to nursing or do something else. Other times, this unfortunate reality must be presented in the form of bad grades or poor clinical evaluations. Nurse Anesthetists have their patients' lives in their hands. It's a great privilege that can't be simply given away...it must be earned. I hope you have what it takes to earn that privilege.

I know I don't have any golden tickets, but hopefully I have provided you with some valuable insight into the life of a CRNA student. I sometimes wish I could have blacked out much of what happened during my 28 months of training. But then I wouldn't be the CRNA I am today and I would have nothing to share with you. I made some great friends and learned a lot about myself. Don't be afraid to make your own mistakes, but try to learn as much as you can from the ones I made.

28-36 months probably seems like forever away. But you won't believe how fast it will go by. It's true that time flies when you're having fun. But it goes by even faster when you're too busy to realize that you're not having any fun at all. Keep your eye on the prize at the end of this long and arduous journey. Whenever you feel like quitting, just remember what you'll have if you choose to forge on. When that day comes, I'll be happy to call you my colleague.

Made in the USA
San Bernardino, CA
13 December 2017